Stress Releaser

S-T-R-E-T-C-H-C-L-O-T-H

Stress Releaser

S·T·R·E·T·C·H·C·L·O·T·H

The gentle way to physical fitness

Lilian Jarvis

PHOTOGRAPHS BY
Andrew Oxenham

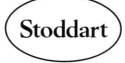
Stoddart

STRESS RELEASER S-T-R-E-T-C-H-C-L-O-T-H™
is a trademark of Moulin Publishing and Lilian Jarvis

Published in 1998 by Stoddart Publishing Co. Limited
34 Lesmill Road, Toronto, Canada M3B 2T6
180 Varick Street, 9th Floor, New York, New York 10014

First published in trade paperback in 1994 by Moulin Publishing Limited

Distributed in Canada by:
General Distribution Services Ltd.
325 Humber College Blvd., Toronto, Ontario M9W 7C3
Tel. (416) 213-1919   Fax (416) 213-1917
Email customer.service@ccmailgw.genpub.com

Distributed in the United States by:
General Distribution Services Inc.
85 River Rock Drive, Suite 202, Buffalo, New York 14207
Toll-free tel. 1-800-805-1083   Toll-free fax 1-800-481-6207
Email gdsinc@genpub.com

02 01 00 99 98   2 3 4 5

Canadian Cataloguing in Publication Data

Jarvis, Lilian, 1931–
Stress releaser S-T-R-E-T-C-H-C-L-O-T-H: the gentle way to physical fitness

Accompanied by a stretch cloth.
ISBN 0-7737-6004-0

1. Stretching exercises.   2. Physical fitness for women.
3. Physical fitness for the aged.   4. Physical fitness for the physically handicapped.
I. Title.

RA781.63.J37 1998   613.7'1   C98-931117-5

Printed and bound in Canada

*Stoddart Publishing gratefully acknowledges the Canada Council for the Arts and
the Ontario Arts Council for their support of our publishing program.*

The exercises and instructions in this book are not intended as a substitute for proper medical advice.
The use of the STRESS RELEASER S-T-R-E-T-C-H-C-L-O-T-H and the stretch exercises
is a personal decision at the sole discretion and risk of the user. Consult your physician
before beginning this or any new exercise program if you have serious concerns
about a negative impact of the exercises on your physical condition.

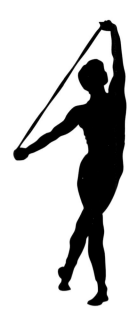

Table of Contents

Introduction 9

The Stretchcloth 11

Working With The Stretchcloth 12

How To Use The Stretchcloth 16

Stress Releaser Exercises

1   Neck, Shoulder, and Back Stretch 18

2   Shoulder and Chest Stretch 20

3   Back Strengthening 22

4   Arm Stretch 24

5   Wrist and Arm Stretches 26

6   Shoulder and Upper Arm Stretch (1) 28

7   Shoulder and Upper Arm Stretch (2) 30

8   Hamstring Stretch 32

9   Lower Back Stretch (1) 34

10   Lower Back Strengthening 36

11   Back Strengthening and Leg Stretch 38

12   Groin and Inner Thigh Stretch 40

13   Abdominal Strengthening (1) 42

14   Abdominal Strengthening (2) 44

15   Hamstring and Groin Stretch 46

16   Inner Thigh Stretch 48

17   Full Body Stretch 50

18   Full Spine and Back Stretch 52

19   Shoulder Stretch .54

20   Upper Back Contraction 56

21   Shoulder Rotation 58

22   Arm Strengthening 60

23   Thigh Stretch 62

24   Spine Rotation 64

25   Stretching and Strengthening the Torso . . .66

26   Lower Back Stretch (2) 68

27   Total Body Relaxation 70

Acknowledgements 72

For several months
now I have been
stretching whatever
wants to be
stretched, making
up how I do it as
I go along, letting
my muscles and
joints tell me
what they need,
doing it whenever
and for as long
as it feels good.
The effect, especially
as compared to routine
body-tightening calisthenics,
is so mentally releasing
that I believe it
somehow nourishes
my psyche, just as eating
exactly what my stomach
tells me it wants
nourishes my flesh.

Hugh Prather

Introduction

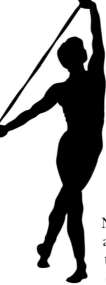

Were it not for an inborn sense of musicality and a heart and soul that longed to dance, I would not have been a principal dancer of Canada's National Ballet through the fifties and early sixties. We were chosen then more for quality and characterization than for having the right kind of body — and mine certainly wasn't. My back was swayed and my hip joints were frustratingly tight, so I could never manage the Charlie Chaplin "turnout" that ballet demanded, nor could I get my legs up much past my hips. It seemed flexibility would be forever beyond my reach. Yet now, many long years later, I can say it's my greatest joy.

At age sixty-three flexibility is what keeps me feeling young and able to move however I want or need to. I can bend, turn, reach and curl up without pain or constraint, walk with fluid ease and still dance if I want to. Being flexible has shown me, too, that the way to a strong and healthy body is through ridding my muscles of tension. More than that, it's what helps me deal with the many stresses that are part of everyday life. What can compare with that kind of mental and bodily freedom?

Whether I was born with my particular tightnesses or had developed them by the time I was thirteen when my ballet training began, I don't know. At any rate, it was only after I came upon an entirely new way of thinking about my body, at the belated age of thirty-three, that I began to understand both the importance of flexibility and how to achieve it. It not only changed the course of my life, it ultimately gave me a new understanding of what it means to be fit.

The seed was planted in 1963 at the Martha Graham School of modern dance. It was there that my eyes were opened to a realm of my body I had never before considered — my inside! The focus of my past training had been on "line," "placing," and "form," all external concepts. Now I was being told to *feel the sensation* of my muscles working — that this was how you got "in touch" with your body and controlled it! Well! That was all I needed. Maybe, I thought, if I got in touch with enough muscles I could finally *do* something about those stubborn hip joints. So, with a fervour bordering on obsession, I began to explore this new-found and mysterious inner realm.

Marriage, and the birth of a child, threatened to thwart my latest ambition. But the compulsion to change my body would not let me rest. For thirteen years my bedroom served as an experimental station where I spent two or three hours a day getting into strange positions and discovering muscles I never knew I had. Some needed to be stretched, while others were weak and needed strengthening. And as the years passed, I found I could not only "feel" them, I could also "see" them as an intricate network that connected the parts of my body. It was like "coming alive" inside!

The long sessions left me exhausted, yet after a few moments of rest I was filled with a kind of energy unlike anything I'd felt before. And the thought would occur to me, "*Now* I'm ready for a dance class!"

The reward for my years of solitary effort came when I returned to the National to dance the role of Juliet for the company's 25th anniversary production of *Romeo and Juliet.* Imperceptibly over the years, my body *had* changed. The sway back was all but gone, my legs were looser, and I felt a strength and vitality that imbued me with delight. After such a long "retirement," the comeback was proof enough for me that I had stumbled onto something pretty great — a wonderful new way to keep fit!

Though I had no system to speak of, I began to teach my self-evolved exercises to anyone who was looking for a way to a better body without the rigours of aerobics. For a number of reasons, the first year I taught was a particularly stressful one, yet it revealed perhaps the most surprising consequence of my unorthodox methods: their effect on reducing stress. I would go to teach my classes in a state of emotional turmoil, yet when they had finished it was as though I hadn't a care in the world. It was hard to believe that the slow stretching and strengthening could make such a difference to my frame of mind, and to this day it amazes me that the after effect is always one of refreshment and tranquillity.

As the exercises became more developed and refined, a simple device completed the evolution of the program. It was the Stretchcloth. This was something I'd come upon quite by accident and found it produced a sensation of stretch that, while intense, was deeply satisfying. I tried it out in classes to see if it affected others the same way, and it was an immediate success. Everyone thought it was *great*. Over the years, the Stretchcloth provided new ways to stretch the legs, arms, shoulders, neck, back, and hands, while bringing a heightened focus to strengthening the more internal parts of the body and hastening the process of discovery I'd gone through myself years before.

Now that you have found it, I hope that the Stretchcloth will help you discover your body in as exciting a way as I discovered mine, and that you too will experience the gratification and pleasure that it's possible to have when your body feels free, flexible and alive!

The S·T·R·E·T·C·H·C·L·O·T·H

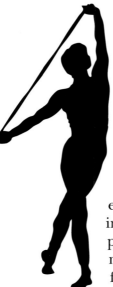

Despite its simplicity, the Stress Releaser Stretchcloth that comes with this book is one of the most helpful exercise aids you'll ever find. It has become an important part of my exercise program, which is based on making your body work better from a "mechanical," as opposed to a cardiovascular, point of view. The exercises increase flexibility through stretching muscles as well as joints, strengthen the deep, skeletal muscles that support your weight, and, ultimately, realign your posture so you stand taller and straighter. The results of this work affect the well-being of both body and mind in ways that are unmistakable.

The first step in this process involves releasing the tension that is locked up in tight muscles. Often this tension is so ingrained that normal exercise doesn't reach it and you may not even know it's there. But it's what limits your normal range of movement and, therefore, limits what you can do with your body.

Much of my flexibility I credit to the kind of Stretchcloth exercises that are in this book. I use them not only in my classes but also for a quick workout each morning. There's nothing that prepares me better for the day. I don't do any sports and I don't jog or lift weights. I scarcely get out to walk. But I feel strong and have few aches, pains, or physiological problems. Moreover, with much of my time now spent at the computer, I can sit for long hours without tiring and without the muscular traumas that this sedentary lifestyle seems to inflict on so many others. I consider myself fortunate indeed.

Though the Stretchcloth is just a long piece of stretchy material, it both stretches and strengthens your body in ways that are impossible without it. It uses your relaxed body weight along with resistance so you can stretch more deeply without straining and without using force. And it strengthens you in a focused way, making you conscious of muscles you were never aware of before. The combined effect of stretching, releasing tension, and internal strengthening gives you a sense of renewed vitality and leaves you feeling relaxed, worked, and energized, all at the same time.

The beauty of the Stretchcloth is that it's like having your own personal gym that you can use wherever you are. You can tuck it into a drawer or suit-case and use it at work or take it with you on trips. It can be easily shortened or lengthened to accommodate your own body tightnesses, and also to take you further into your body as you become more flexible.

What the Stretchcloth exercises can mean to you is a more supple, stronger, and straighter body, less tension, fewer aches and pains, strains or injuries, better physiological health, and increased stamina for other activities. Even a small increase in flexibility, whatever your age, will help reduce your level of stress, stimulate your inner "workings," and minimize that insidious stiffening that creeps up on us all over the years.

To get the best results from the exercises, be sure to read the section Working With the Stretchcloth as well as the instructions on How to Use the Stretchcloth before you begin working with it.

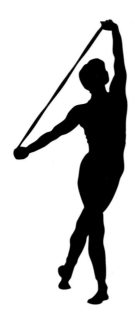

Working With the
S~T~R~E~T~C~H~C~L~O~T~H

Working with the Stretchcloth will stretch your mind as well as your muscles. The exercises are unique in that they require *opposing pressures* within your body. That is, one part of your body "presses" in one direction while another part presses the opposite way. This means that you have to think in two, and sometimes three, different directions at the same time.

This is not something our linear minds are accustomed to. They tend to think in only one direction at a time, and changing this takes concentration. But that's what makes the process so absorbing. It's how you "get in touch" with your body and how you can become confident that you *are* in control of it. Once you've reached this stage, you'll never again see your body and mind as having separate functions. They'll work in harmony together, not as your body *and* your mind, but as one "you."

S~T~R~E~T~C~H~C~L~O~T~H

Something else that's different about the Stretchcloth exercises is the use of your *abdominal muscles*, and it relates partly to the rule of thumb for breathing, which is: *always breathe in before you start an exercise and breathe out as you do the exercise.* In breathing out, the abdominal muscles work much like a bellows, which forces air out in a continuous stream when its two sides are pushed together. In the same way, when you draw your abdomen in, your breath is forced steadily out of your lungs. This allows you to do the exercises without creating tension throughout your body.

The feeling to aim for as you breathe out is a gradual pulling in of your abdomen toward your spine, with the strongest pull at the centre of your waist, right at your belly button. Then, when you let go of your muscles, air will automatically be drawn into your lungs, just as it's drawn into a bellows when the sides open. As you learn to work your abdominal muscles this way, your breathing will become a coordinated part of the exercises and not something you have to think about. (For brevity, the abdominal muscles are referred to in the exercises simply as "your abdominals.")

S~T~R~E~T~C~H~C~L~O~T~H

As well as controlling your breathing, your abdominal muscles are used in each exercise with varying strength depending on their purpose. Where you read, *draw your abdominals in lightly,* the purpose is simply to hold your pelvis straight. This is how you should be before you begin an exercise, whether sitting or standing. *Draw your abdominals in* means actively pulling them in to prevent your lower back from arching during the exercise. Where using your abdominals is vital to the exercise, such as to create pressure against your spine, you'll find *draw your abdominals in strongly.*

S-T-R-E-T-C-H-C-L-O-T-H

The *deep breath* that you take to begin each exercise is to ensure that you have enough air so you can breathe out continuously for the duration of the exercise. If you think of this first breath as the beginning of a big sigh, that should fill your lungs sufficiently. Taking a deep breath at the end of an exercise helps to release tension. This breath is the kind that happens after a long, deep stretch or extended effort, and it will generally happen naturally if you let it. You can, of course, also take a deep breath whenever you feel the need.

S-T-R-E-T-C-H-C-L-O-T-H

Press is used to mean directional pressure and does not involve tightening your muscles. For example, pressing your hands outward into the cloth when your hands are overhead should produce the same feeling in your arms as if your hands were pressing gently against a wall on either side of you. Similarly, *pull on the cloth* involves no "gripping" of your arms or shoulders. The only grip is in your hands, and just enough to hold the cloth firmly.

S-T-R-E-T-C-H-C-L-O-T-H

Press your chest forward refers only to your upper chest. The pressure comes from contracting your shoulder blades and pressing them forward. If you're breathing out and your abdominal muscles are drawn in, your lower ribs should not open nor your lower back overarch.

S-T-R-E-T-C-H-C-L-O-T-H

The words *hold* and *stay with* are purposely used in place of "hold the position," which is static and does not apply to these exercises. Although you'll notice no changes in the external appearance of your body during the "hold" time, the muscles you're using continue to "press" or "pull."

S-T-R-E-T-C-H-C-L-O-T-H

Suggesting how many times to do an exercise or how long to hold a stretch has also been purposely avoided. Everyone's body is different, and what is too much stretch or is too exhausting for one person is not enough for another. *Judging your own limits* is part of getting to know your body, and this will help you know how much to push yourself in more strenuous activities as well.

S-T-R-E-T-C-H-C-L-O-T-H

When you begin these exercises, don't try to copy the photos exactly. They show an advanced state of flexibility and your ultimate goal. It takes time to become flexible, and the best way to do that is by degrees. Tailor the exercises to your own capabilities and *let your body tell you when it's ready to go further.*

S-T-R-E-T-C-H-C-L-O-T-H

You'll find the active part of the exercises — when you're breathing out — is broken into separate sentences to make the instructions easier for you to follow, but all of the exercises are meant to be done as *one smooth and continuous movement*. When you feel familiar with what each part of your body is doing, work toward synchronizing the different movements, or pressures, so they happen at the same time.

S-T-R-E-T-C-H-C-L-O-T-H

Remember always to *do the exercises slowly*, both going in and coming out of them. And stop an exercise if you feel a sharp pain. It may be nothing serious, but it *is* a warning sign that you've found a weakness or some other problem that requires caution. The solution often is simply to do the exercise more gently, but if the sharpness persists, have it checked by your doctor or chiropractor. If you should experience some nausea, lie down for a while and breathe deeply. Though it's not uncommon, this reaction will stop once your body adjusts to the deeper work.

S-T-R-E-T-C-H-C-L-O-T-H

As with any exercise that is new to you, you may experience some stiffness in the beginning, so I suggest you start with only a few exercises and spread the rest out over the following days. Then *concentrate on your "problem" areas*. Do the first three exercises, for example, any time your back and shoulders feel tired and achy. And pick out the ones you need to work with most — the ones you find "difficult." That will help you work through your major blocks. For an overall workout the exercises are laid out in a sequence that works in a natural progression through your body, so simply follow the order given. Try to finish each session with Exercise 27 regardless of whether you work through the whole set. It's a wonderfully relaxing "non-exercise."

Don't worry if you don't *feel* an exercise where you think you "should." Although they're focused on specific parts of the body, they all affect more than one area, so use them to your own best advantage. When you can't do exactly what the instructions say because of some physical restriction, do the exercise as best you can, but keep the goal in mind so you can work toward it if at all possible, now or later.

S-T-R-E-T-C-H-C-L-O-T-H

Once you're comfortable with the exercises, feel free to experiment. The ones here are just examples of how the Stretchcloth can be used, but many other variations are possible. Try changing the height or angle of your arms, for example, or moving your body in different ways while you create resistance with the cloth. Every small change you make will register differently "inside." Becoming aware of those sensations is what discovering your body is all about.

S-T-R-E-T-C-H-C-L-O-T-H

Exercises 1 to 8 are shown sitting because they're ones you can do while working at a desk and because it's less tiring for your legs than doing many exercises standing. However, except for Exercise 8, they can be done standing as well. Conversely, Exercises 21 and 22 can be done sitting.

S-T-R-E-T-C-H-C-L-O-T-H

Note that in the instructions, *cloth length* refers to the length that's left between your hands after you've wrapped the cloth around them. In all exercises, your hands stay lightly closed on the cloth unless otherwise specified.

S-T-R-E-T-C-H-C-L-O-T-H

Finally, with so many demands on daily life, it's easy to short change the most important person in your life — you! So try to find some special times when you can go through all the exercises. Find a space of your own and put on some mellow music to help slow you down, then devote this time to yourself. I can assure you your body will thank you for it!

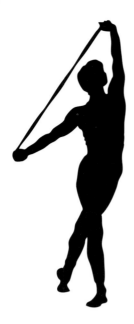

How to Use the
S·T·R·E·T·C·H·C·L·O·T·H

Using the Stretchcloth is easy once you get a feel for handling it. Wrapping it properly around your hands is a good place to start. Here's how you do it:

1. Hold one end of the cloth in your right hand, palm facing down, with the end toward your little finger.

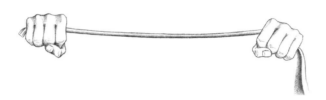

2. With your left hand, wrap the cloth clockwise around the palm of your right hand three or four times, with the end secured underneath the wrapped layers.
Scrunch the cloth together as you're wrapping it so it doesn't cover your hand like a bandage.

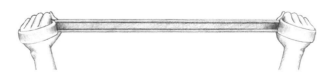

3. Slide your left hand along the cloth to the other end and wrap the cloth clockwise around your left palm. Then pull outward with both hands so the cloth is snug around both palms.

You should now have about 1 metre (3 feet) of cloth between your hands, which is a good length for many of the exercises. However, some need less than that and some need more. The length of your arms and your degree of tightness will also determine how long your cloth should be.

You can easily adjust the length to suit you. To make the cloth longer, simply unwrap a loop or two from either hand. Or add more loops to shorten it. You can also make smaller adjustments by wrapping the last loop around only the first two fingers of one hand or of both hands. If you prefer, you can circle your hands into the cloth with the ends hanging free — as long as you don't mind them flapping around your head in some exercises.

In most of the stretching exercises, you need to transfer weight from your body into the Stretchcloth in order to relax your muscles. To see how this works, try the following test which transfers the weight of your arms into the cloth:

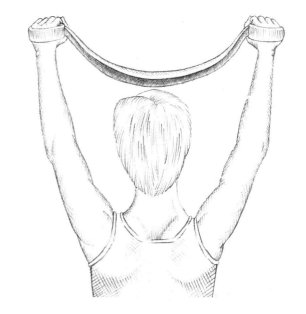

1. Wrap the cloth snugly around both palms, as instructed, leaving a good 1 metre (3 feet) between them. Then raise your arms overhead so the cloth is positioned above your head. The cloth should be slack, as shown.

2. Hold the cloth lightly and press your hands out to both sides until the cloth is tight. Then relax your hands, shoulders, and arms, letting your arms drop backward from your shoulders a little. (You may have to make the cloth longer if your shoulders are tight.) The cloth, in effect, will now be holding your arms up, with the weight of each arm balancing the other. Your shoulders will be "dropped" and you'll feel the cloth pressing against the outside edges of your hands. (If you find it difficult to relax your shoulders, try taking a deep breath then dropping your shoulders suddenly and letting your breath out at the same time. Then try doing it more gradually.)

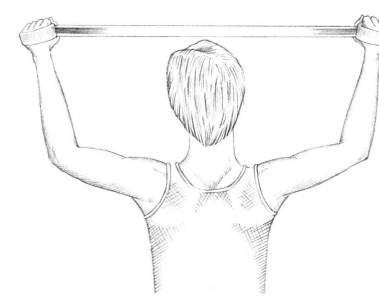

3. Now use your muscles to hold your arms up. The cloth will again be slack.

If you do this sequence slowly several times, you'll feel your arm and shoulder muscles alternately relaxing and gripping as weight is transferred from your arms into the cloth and back to your arms again. The relaxed feeling in your muscles — "letting go" of them — is what you want. In some exercises this allows gravity to exert a downward pull on the muscles. In others your muscles are stretched more intensely by pressing against resistance from the cloth.

Keep in mind that stretching always produces a "pulled" sensation, so don't mistake the feeling you get from a stretch with not being relaxed. As long as you're not tensing or "holding" your muscles, they're as relaxed as they can be. "Using" your muscles always produces a sensation of tightening, or gripping, which is quite different from the pulled sensation of a stretch.

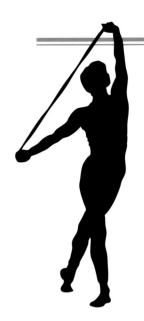

1 Neck, Shoulder, and Back Stretch

This is a good exercise to do whenever your neck, shoulders, and back feel tired and achy. If you do it on a regular basis, it will help prevent the build-up of tension.

Cloth length— about 0.6 metre (2 feet)

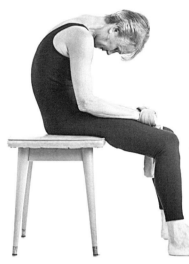

1◀ Breathing normally, lower your head slowly forward and relax your neck muscles. Then slowly relax your body, letting your back round out, your chest cave in, and your shoulders droop.

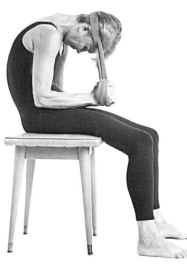

2◀ When you're fully relaxed, place the cloth across the back of your head, just above your ears. Lower your hands and relax your shoulders so your hands hang down. Then press down gently on the cloth to increase the stretch to your neck, shoulders, and back. If that feels too intense, just let your arms hang.

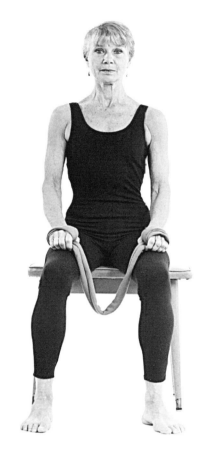

▲ Sit on a chair with your back erect and your arms down with the cloth between your hands, with your feet and knees spaced comfortably apart. Rest your hands on your thighs. Take a deep breath in, lifting your shoulders and filling your lungs completely, then breathe out through your mouth as your shoulders come down. (This exercise can be done sitting or standing.)

3 Stay with the stretch as long as you're comfortable. Then take the cloth off your head, rest your hands on your thighs, and slowly straighten your spine, bringing your head up last. Take another complete breath, circle your shoulders to loosen your back, then sink slowly into the relaxed position again and place the cloth across the back of your head.

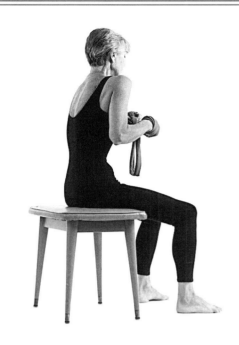

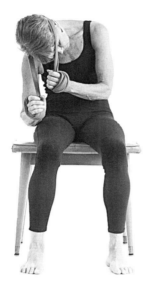

4◄ With your shoulders relaxed and your hands hanging down, roll your head slowly so it leans toward your right shoulder. Stay with the stretch, feeling the pull to the left side of your neck and back. Then roll your head slowly so it leans toward your left shoulder. Continue rolling your head slowly from side to side, feeling the stretch change across your neck and back.

7▲ Lower your elbows to your sides and circle your shoulders loosely, front to back.

5 When you're ready to come up, centre your body over your hips, take the cloth off your head, and straighten your spine slowly as before.

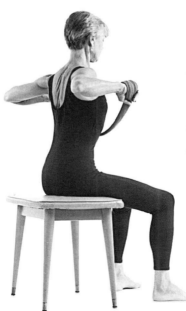

6◄ To counteract the stretch, take a deep breath in as you raise your elbows to both sides, shoulder height. Then breathe out as you press your chest forward and your arms back, contracting your shoulderblades.

Helpful Hints

The aim of this exercise is to relax your muscles completely so the weight of your body pulls on them. It looks simple, but it can feel quite intense. While you need to take time with each step, if at any point the stretch feels too intense, bring yourself slowly out of it, take a breath, and start again. When you feel you can go through the exercise without a break, you can leave out step 3.

Lifting your shoulders when you take a deep breath will allow air to fill your lungs right to the top.

When you're in the relaxed position your shoulders should stay over your hips. You can either let your stomach relax or keep your abdominals lightly drawn in if that's more comfortable.

Don't lift your shoulders or arms when your head rolls from side to side. Leave them relaxed so they stay below your head. Let your hands move up and down with the cloth as it lengthens on one side and shortens on the other.

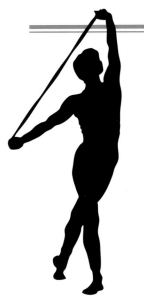

2 Shoulder and Chest Stretch

Besides relieving daily fatigue, this exercise is great to do in the morning to relieve night-time stiffness. It stretches your shoulders, opens your chest, and contracts your back muscles.

Cloth length — 1 metre (3 feet)
or longer if your shoulders are tight

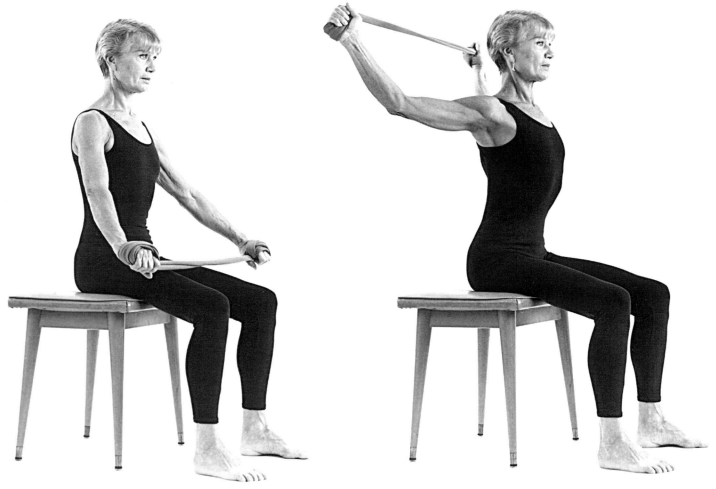

▲ **S**it on a chair with your back erect, feet and knees comfortably apart, and arms down with the cloth straight between your hands. (This exercise can be done sitting or standing.)

1 Take a deep breath in as you circle your arms overhead.

2▲ As you breathe out, draw your abdominals in and press both hands outward, stretching the cloth. Then press your chest forward and contract your shoulder blades as you press your arms back. Tilt your head down to relax your neck.

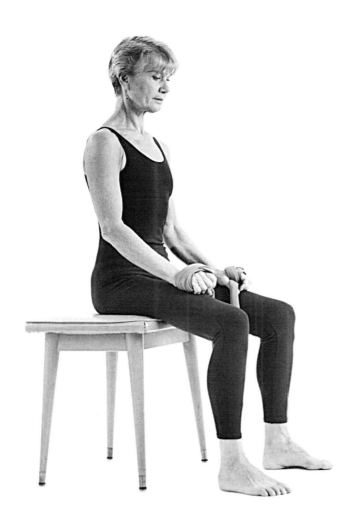

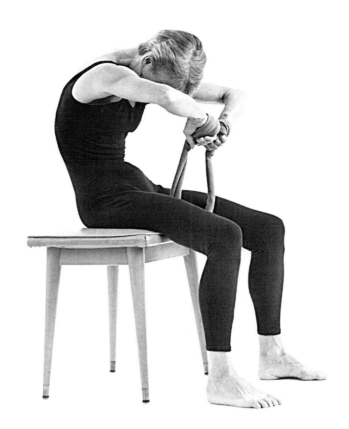

3▲ Hold while you feel the stretch in your shoulders and chest. Then, breathing as necessary, bring your arms forward and relax them down.

4 Repeat from step 1 several times.

5▲ To stretch your back when you've finished, lower your head and pull your arms and shoulders strongly forward as you round your back and press it out.

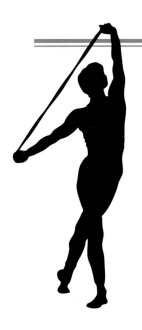

3 Back Strengthening

Another good exercise to relieve your tired back, this one also opens the chest and helps you get a good grip on the upper back muscles so you can straighten your back.

Cloth length — at least 1 metre (3 feet)

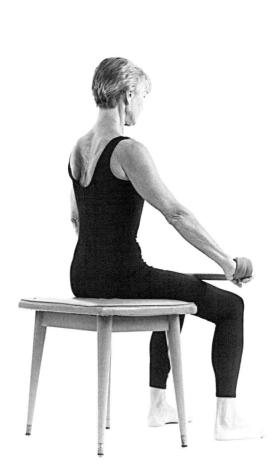

▲ **S**it on a chair with your back erect, feet and knees comfortably apart, and your arms down with the cloth straight between your hands. (This exercise can be done sitting or standing.)

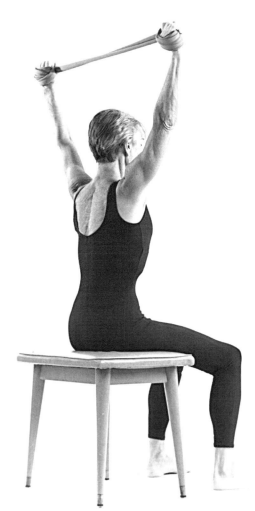

1 ▲ Take a deep breath in as you lift your arms straight overhead.

3 ◄ Keep your chin level and your hands pressed out to both sides while you feel the contraction in your back. Then take a deep breath in as you lift your arms up, relaxing your pull on the cloth.

4 Repeat from step 2 several times.

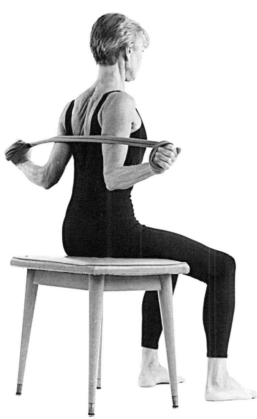

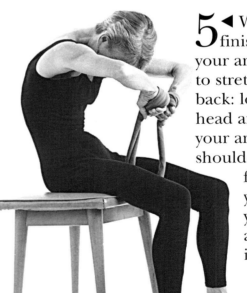

2 ▲ As you breathe out, draw your abdominals in and press your hands out to both sides so the cloth is tight, then relax your arms and shoulders.* Bring the cloth down your back, bending your elbows to your sides until the cloth is in a straight line behind your shoulders.

5 ◄ When you've finished, bring your arms in front to stretch your back: lower your head and pull your arms and shoulders strongly forward as you round your back and press it out.

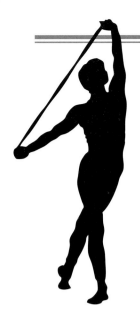

4 Arm Stretch

This stretch releases deep tension from your arms. It stretches the muscles on the inside of your arms, loosens your shoulder joints, and opens your chest. With your head tilted, it stretches the side of your neck as well.

Cloth length— at least 1 metre (3 feet)

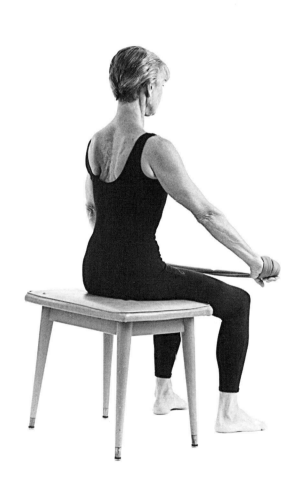

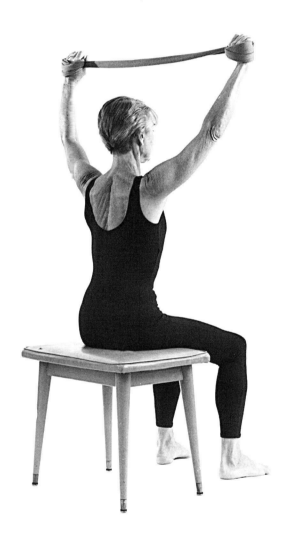

▲ **S**it on a chair with your back erect, feet and knees comfortably apart, and your arms down with the cloth straight between your hands. (This exercise can be done sitting or standing.)

1 ▲ Take a deep breath in as you circle your arms overhead.

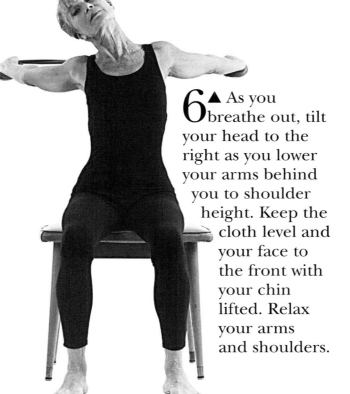

6▲ As you breathe out, tilt your head to the right as you lower your arms behind you to shoulder height. Keep the cloth level and your face to the front with your chin lifted. Relax your arms and shoulders.

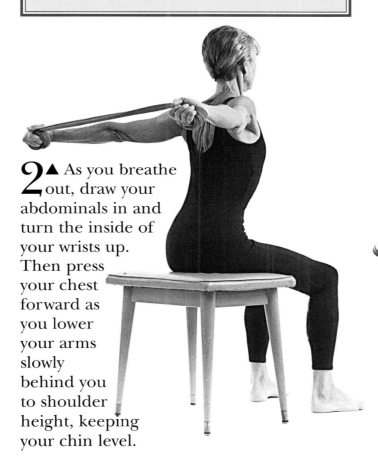

2▲ As you breathe out, draw your abdominals in and turn the inside of your wrists up. Then press your chest forward as you lower your arms slowly behind you to shoulder height, keeping your chin level.

3 Hold while you feel the stretch through your arms and chest. Then, breathing as necessary, bring your arms forward and relax them down.

4 Repeat from step 1 several times. Then go on to step 5.

5 Take a deep breath in as you circle your arms overhead.

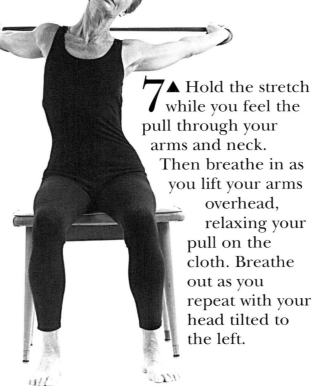

7▲ Hold the stretch while you feel the pull through your arms and neck. Then breathe in as you lift your arms overhead, relaxing your pull on the cloth. Breathe out as you repeat with your head tilted to the left.

8 Repeat to each side at least once more. Bring your arms down to finish.

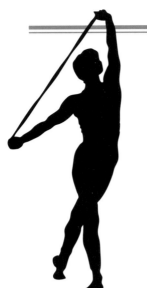

5 Wrist and Arm Stretches

These stretches release tension from your arms. You'll feel the first one through the length of your arm right into your first two fingers. The second one stretches through the back of your wrists and the outside of your lower arms. Make sure you go into both slowly!

> **Cloth length — at least 0.6 metre (2 feet)**
> with the last wrap around the first two fingers of each hand.

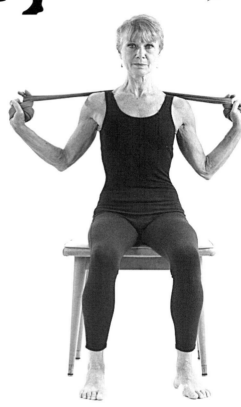
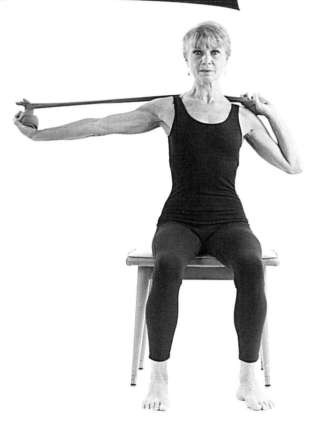

▲ **S**it on a chair with your back erect, feet and knees comfortably apart and your arms with the cloth straight between your hands. Lift the cloth over your head and place it across your shoulders. Take a deep breath in. (This exercise can be done sitting or standing.)

1 ▲ As you breathe out, draw your abdominals in lightly and slowly straighten your right arm to the side so the wrist and first two fingers are bent and pulled back. Then tighten your arm. If you need to, move your left hand toward, or away from, your shoulder so the cloth is tight when your arm is straight.

Helpful Hints

In the first stretch, bend your elbow a little if there's too much pull on your wrist. Pressing your shoulder down gently after you tighten your arm will increase the stretch.

In the second stretch, relax your shoulders if the pull on your wrists is not too intense.

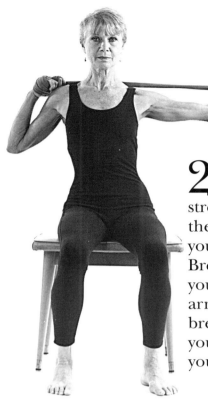

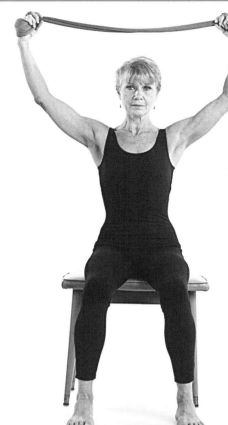

2 ◄ Hold while you feel the stretch through the length of your arm. Breathe in as you change arms, and breathe out as you straighten your left arm.

4 ◄ Take a deep breath in as you raise your arms above your head, elbows bent, palms turned down, and your fingers holding the cloth lightly.

5 As you breathe out, press both wrists gently to each side so the cloth is slightly stretched. Tilt your head forward to relax your neck.

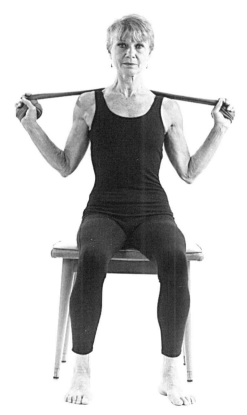

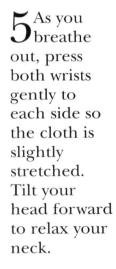

6 ◄ Feel the stretch through the back of your wrists and lower arms. Then breathe in as you lift your arms a little to release the stretch.

3 ▲ Repeat from step 2 several times. Then centre the cloth behind your shoulders for the second stretch.

7 Repeat from step 5 several times. When you've finished, relax your arms down.

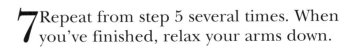

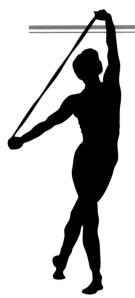

6 Shoulder and Upper Arm Stretch (1)

This exercise stretches your upper arm muscles and increases the flexibility of your shoulder joints so you can lift your arms straight overhead.

Cloth length — about 0.6 metre (2 feet)

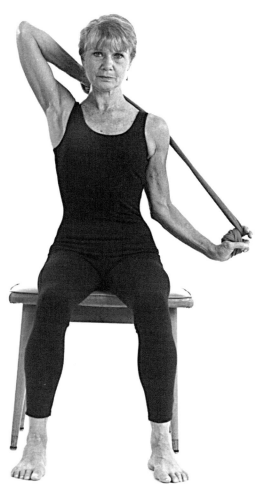

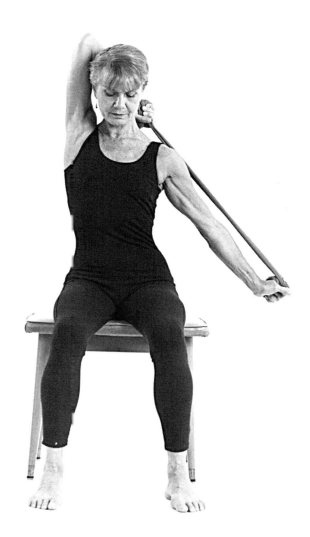

▲ **S**it on a chair with your back erect, feet and knees comfortably apart, and your arms down with the cloth straight between your hands. Lift your right hand over your head and rest it on the back of your neck. Leave your left arm at your side. Take a deep breath in.

1 ▲ As you breathe out, draw your abdominals in while you press your left arm slowly to the side so your right elbow is pulled toward the ceiling. Tilt your head forward and let your hand slide past your neck. Try to relax your shoulder.

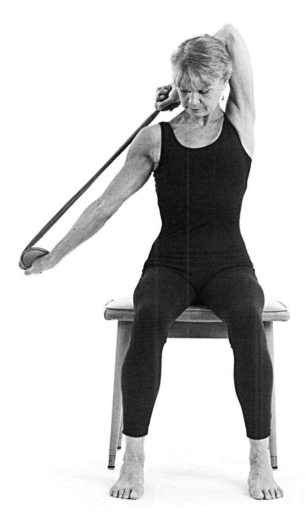

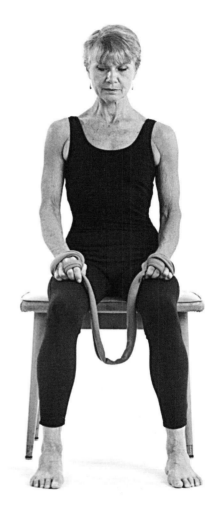

2▲ Breathe normally while you hold, feeling the stretch in your shoulder and arm. Then breathe in as you reverse your arms, and breathe out as you stretch the left.

3▲ Repeat to both sides several times. When you've finished, relax your arms down.

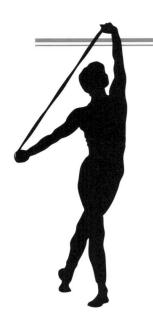

7 Shoulder and Upper Arm Stretch (2)

The Stretchcloth makes this exercise an easier version of the yoga stretch in which the hands clasp each other behind the back. You'll feel the stretch in the front of your shoulder and upper arm muscles.

Cloth length — about 0.6 metre (2 feet)

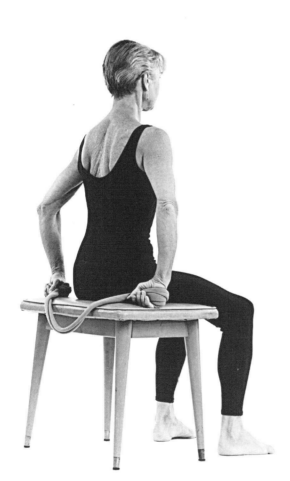

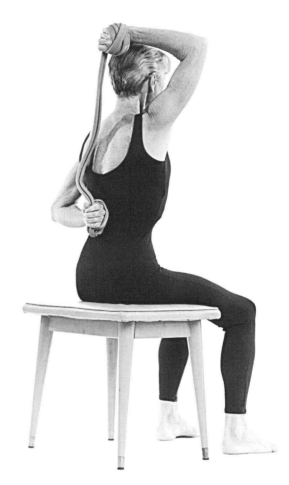

▲ **S**it on a chair with your back erect, feet and knees comfortably apart. Take the cloth behind you and wrap it around your hands until they're at both sides of your hips, palms facing back. (This exercise can be done sitting or standing.)

1 ▲ Place the back of your left hand against your lower back. Holding your right elbow out, circle your right hand toward you and bring it forward over the cloth. Then bring your elbow forward as well. Place your hand at the back of your head and take a deep breath in.

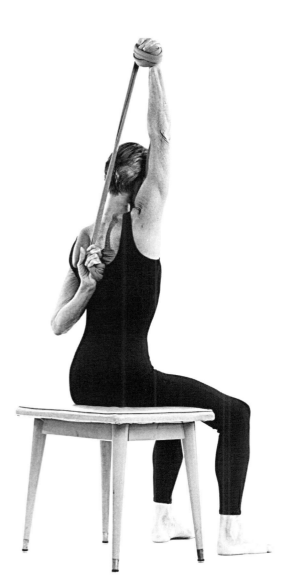

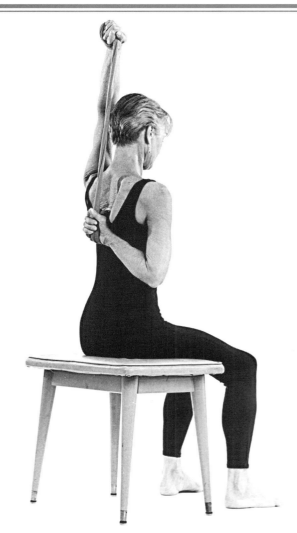

2▲ As you breathe out, draw your abdominals in and pull your right hand slowly up so the left hand is drawn up your back. Tilt your head forward to relax your neck.

3 Breathe normally while you hold, feeling the stretch in your shoulder and arm. Then breathe in as you lower your right hand to relax the pull.

4 Repeat from step 2 several times.

5▲ Lower your right hand to the side. Take the left hand off your back and turn both hands toward you at the wrists as you move your hands across to the left. Place your right hand on your back and bring your left hand and elbow forward over the cloth. Place your left hand behind your head and repeat the exercise, stretching your right shoulder and arm.

6 When you've finished, lower your arms behind you and loosen the cloth from your hands.

Helpful Hints

Don't clench your hands. If the cloth is snug around them, they can be relaxed.

Keep the palm of your back hand turned away from you and the arm and shoulder forward.

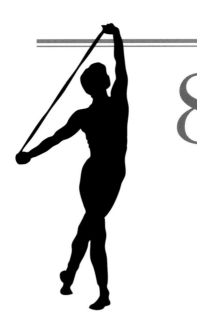

8 Hamstring Stretch

This exercise gives your hamstrings a good stretch and works the muscles in your back at the same time. It's a great one to do after you've been sitting for hours at a desk.

Cloth length — to suit you

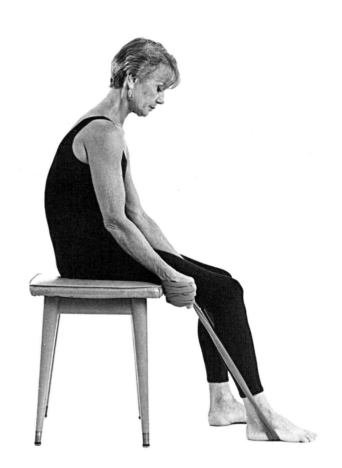

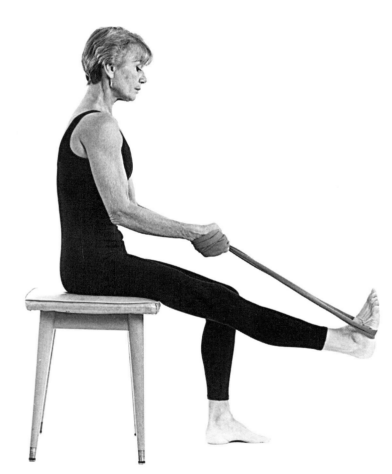

▲ **S**it on a chair. Bend down and slip the middle of the cloth under the sole of your right foot, then slide your hands to the ends as you sit up. Circle your hands into both lengths until your hands are level with your knees. Relax your back.

1 ▲ Take a deep breath in as you straighten your leg, lifting your foot off the floor.

To increase the stretch, pull harder on the cloth and and lean forward from the base of your spine.

Keep the centre of your foot lined up with the shin so your ankle is straight.

As your flexibility improves, lift your thigh off the chair before you straighten your leg. This will make your back work harder.

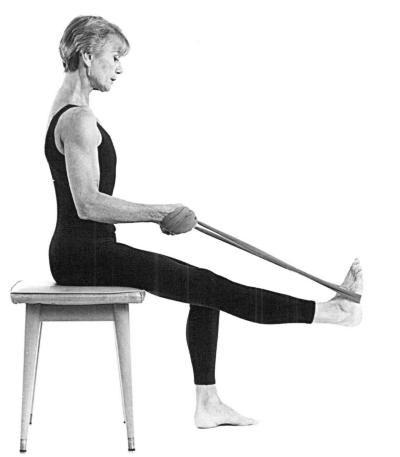

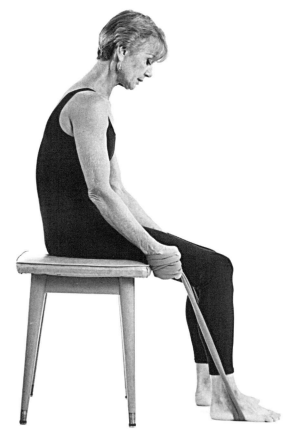

2▲ As you breathe out, draw your abdominals in and pull on the cloth, bending your elbows back toward you. At the same time, straighten your back slowly from the base of your spine.

3▲ Breathe normally while you hold, feeling the stretch through the back of your leg. Then slowly relax your back and lower your foot to the floor.

4 Repeat from step 1 several times. When you've finished, change the cloth to the left foot and repeat the exercise.

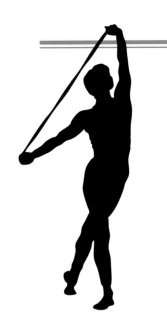

9 Lower Back Stretch (1)

This exercise is a gentle way to stretch out the tight muscles in your lower back and relieve tired achiness.

Cloth Length — about 0.6 metre (2 feet)

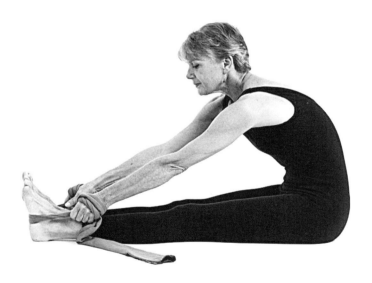

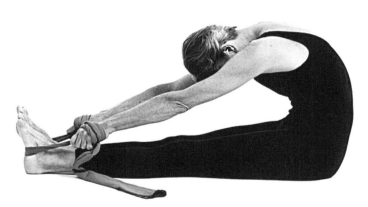

▲ **S**it on the floor, legs in front and feet together. Put the middle of the cloth across the soles of your feet. Take hold of the cloth close to your feet and circle your hands into both lengths a few times, leaving the ends free. Straighten your arms and hold the cloth firmly. Take a deep breath in.

1▲ As you breathe out, draw your abdominals in and lower your head. Leaving your back rounded, pull your body slowly away from your feet and press out through the back of your waist. Keep your arms straight and your shoulders relaxed.

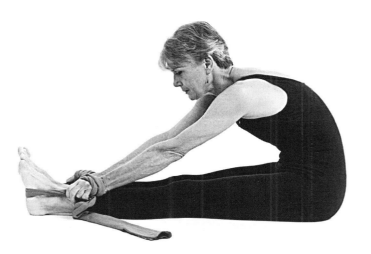

Pull back gently at first so you can evaluate how much pressure your lower back can take. Increase the pressure gradually if you have no sign of discomfort. Remember to have any persistent pain checked by your doctor or chiropractor.

Sometimes lower back muscles are so tight that they don't "give," in which case you may feel this stretch more — or only — in your upper back and shoulders. That's good, too, but keep the focus on your waist.

2▲ Breathe normally while you hold, feeling the stretch in your lower back. Then breathe in as you relax forward.

3 Repeat from step 1 several times.

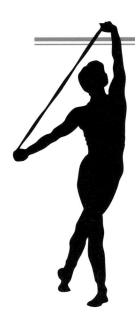

10 Lower Back Strengthening

This exercise strengthens the muscles in the back of your pelvis and loosens your hip joints. It will be especially helpful to you if you find it difficult to sit on the floor with your back straight.

Cloth length — to suit you

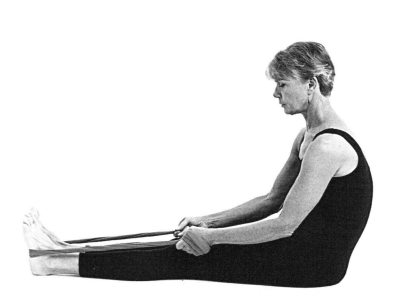

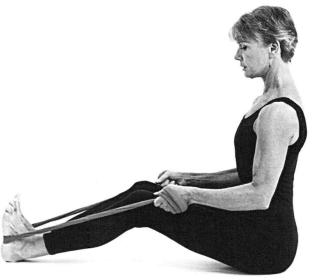

▲ **S**it on the floor with your legs in front and feet together. Put the middle of the cloth across the soles of your feet, then slide your hands along both lengths as you bring your shoulders back over your hips. Circle your hands into the cloth until your hands are level with your knees. Relax your back and take a deep breath in.

1▲ As you breathe out, draw your abdominals in and, without moving your heels, pull on the cloth, flex your ankles, and bend your knees, letting them separate. Continue pulling as you draw your abdominals in more strongly and straighten your back from the base of your spine. Then press the back of your pelvis forward.

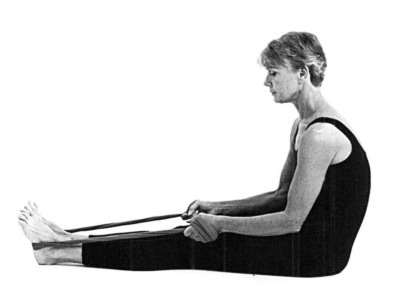

2▲ Hold while you feel the "grip" in your lower back, then breathe in as you slowly relax your muscles.

3 Repeat from step 1 several times.

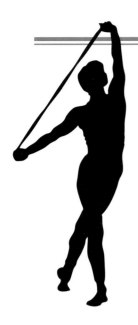

11 Back Strengthening and Leg Stretch

This exercise, like the previous one, loosens your hip joints and strengthens your lower back. But it also strengthens the muscles in your upper back and gives a good stretch to the back of your legs.

Cloth length— to suit you

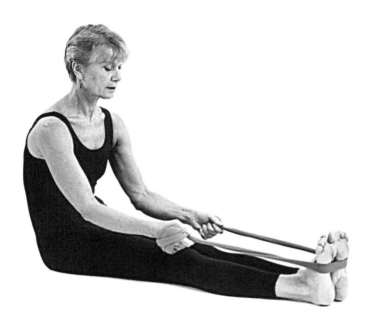

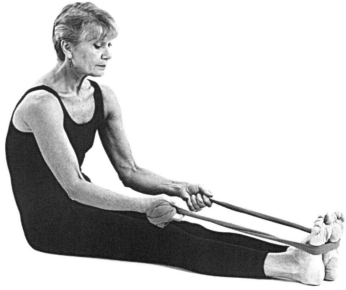

▲ **S**it on the floor with your legs in front and feet together. Put the middle of the cloth across the soles of your feet, then slide your hands along both lengths as you bring your shoulders back over your hips. Circle your hands into the cloth until your hands are level with your knees. Relax your back and take a deep breath in.

1 ▲ As you breathe out, draw your abdominals in, flex your ankles, and pull on the cloth. Continue pulling as you draw your abdominals in more strongly and straighten your back from the base of your spine. Then tighten your legs.

2 Hold while you feel the pull in your legs and back, then breathe in as you slowly relax your muscles.

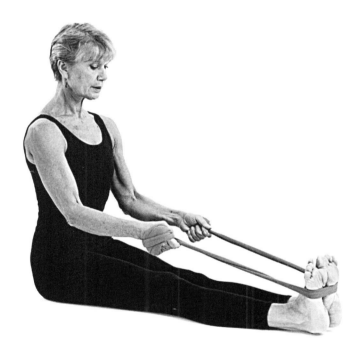

3 ▲ Repeat from step 1 several times. The last time hold the position as long as you can, breathing normally. Then slowly push your heels away, keeping your legs straight.

4 Relax your muscles and take a good deep breath.

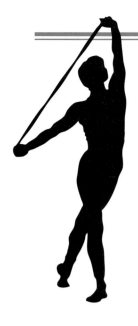

12 Groin and Inner Thigh Stretch

This exercise increases the range of movement in your hip joints. It stretches the inside of your thighs but it's mainly for the groin, an area that most leg stretches don't reach as directly as this one.

Cloth length — to suit you

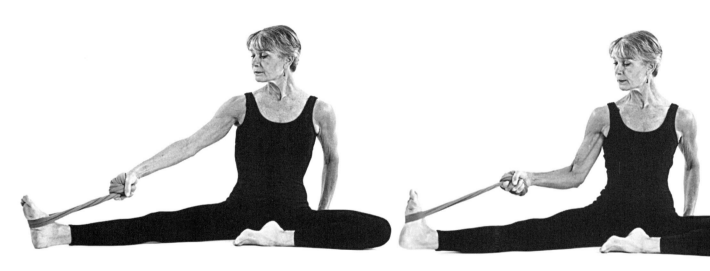

▲ **S**it on the floor. Tuck your left foot in front of your body with the knee dropped out to the side. Open your right leg to the opposite side as far back as possible and put the cloth across the sole of the foot. Hold both ends of the cloth in your right hand and wrap the cloth around it, taking up the slack. Put your left hand on the floor at your side. Straighten your back with your shoulders over your hips and take a deep breath in.

1▲ As you breathe out, draw your abdominals in while you pull on the cloth and tighten your right leg and buttock. Then press your thigh down against the floor.

2 Hold while you feel the stretch to your inner thigh and groin, then breathe in as you relax the muscles.

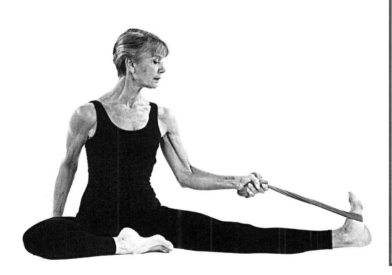

Helpful Hints

This exercise has a strengthening effect on the muscles at the back of your waist. However, it works only one side at a time, so do only 2 or 3 repeats before changing sides. If your back feels uncomfortable, leave the exercise until your back is in better condition.

Both "sit-bones" should be on the floor. If they're not, use the hand that's on the floor to help centre your body, or move the side leg forward a little. Keep your abdominals drawn in throughout to help hold your pelvis upright.

Bend your elbow when you pull on the cloth and leave your shoulder as relaxed as possible.

Flex your ankle and push the heel away to increase the stretch to the back of your leg.

3▲ Repeat from step 1 several times. When you've finished, reverse your leg positions and repeat the exercise with the left leg.

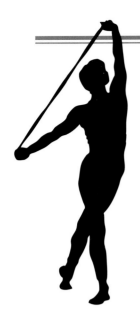

13 Abdominal Strengthening (1)

Strengthening your abdominal muscles will help flatten your stomach and prevent excessive arching in your lower back. You can isolate and strengthen these muscles more effectively when you start from a sitting position.

Cloth length — to suit you

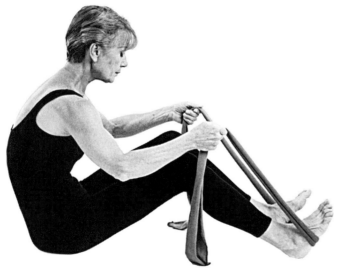

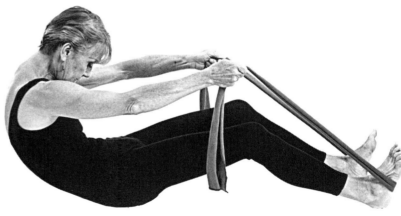

▲ **S**it on the floor with your knees half bent and feet a little wider than hip-width apart. Flex your ankles and put the middle of the cloth across the soles of your feet. Then slide your hands along the cloth as you bring your shoulders back over your hips. Hold the two lengths loosely by your knees, leaving the ends free. Relax your back and take a deep breath in.

1▲ As you breathe out, draw your abdominals in strongly, lower your head, and pull upward on the cloth. In a continuous movement, tip back on your pelvis and lower the back of your waist toward the floor. Keep your back rounded, your shoulders "dropped," and your elbows wide, so the front of your body is "hollowed."

To keep tension out of your thighs, leave them separated as you tip back. That will also help focus your energy into your abdominals. Press the bottom of your pelvis strongly upward so you feel the pull in the muscles just above your pubic bone and in the groin.

If your neck tenses up, you may be pulling your head forward or you've tipped back too far and lost the hold on your abdominals. Think of folding your body at the waist, and lift up on the cloth more to help support your weight.

Try to bring yourself up with your abdominals and use the cloth only as a help. As the muscles strengthen and your back becomes more flexible, you will need the cloth less and less until you can do the exercise without it.

Be sure to lift up on the cloth as you come up. If you pull it toward you you'll create tension through your body and lose the proper effect on your abdominals. Once your shoulders are over the hips you can finish the movement unaided.

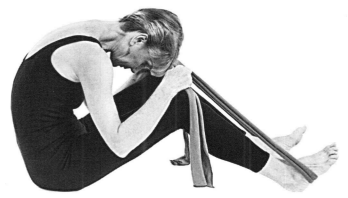

2 ▲ Lift up on the cloth to bring yourself up, keeping your abdominals drawn in and your back rounded. Breathe in as you relax over your knees, bringing your arms down.

3 Repeat from step 1 as many times as your abdominals can stand!

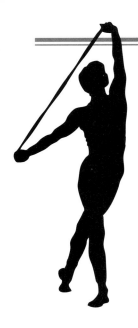

14 Abdominal Strengthening (2)

This is an excellent exercise for strengthening the abdominals when you're able to straighten your legs in the air. When done without the cloth, this exercise usually puts strain on the lower back, but here the cloth prevents strain by supporting your legs as you lower and lift them.

Cloth length — to suit you

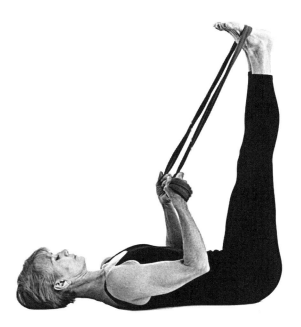

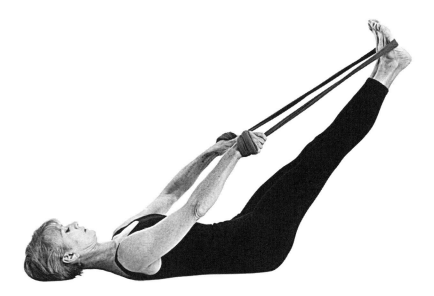

▲ **L**ie on the floor on your back. Bend your knees and put the middle of the cloth across the soles of your feet. Then slide your hands to the ends as you straighten your legs over your hips. Circle your hands into both lengths to take up the slack. Take a deep breath in.

1▲ As you breathe out, draw your abdominals in strongly, then lower your legs slowly past your hips, but only to the point where you feel your waist is *about* to lift.

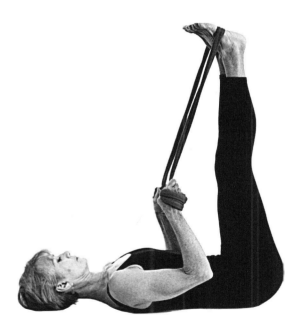

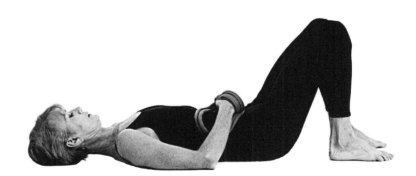

2▲ Hold your legs here until your breath runs out. Then take another deep breath as you pull on the cloth to bring your legs back over your hips.

3▲ Repeat from step 1 as often as you can. When you've finished, bend your knees, remove the cloth, and place your feet, one at a time, on the floor close to your buttocks.

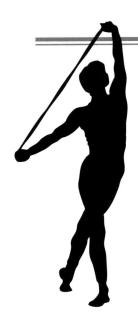

15 Hamstring and Groin Stretch

The secret to stretching hamstrings — whether you're standing, sitting, or lying down — is to bend your hip joints as much as possible while keeping your back straight. This exercise helps you do both and stretches your groin gently as well.

Cloth length — to suit you

▲ Lie on the floor on your back. Leave your left leg relaxed on the floor and bend your right leg over your chest. Put the middle of the cloth across the sole of your right foot, then raise the foot so it's directly above the knee, sole facing the ceiling. Circle your hands into the cloth to take up the slack, then pull down gently on your foot, relaxing the thigh toward your chest. Take a deep breath in.

1 ▲ As you breathe out, draw your abdominals in and pull strongly on the cloth while you slowly straighten your right leg. Tighten the leg, then slowly straighten your left leg to stretch the groin, tightening the thigh and buttock. If you can't straighten your right leg completely, ease up on the cloth and let your arms straighten as necessary.

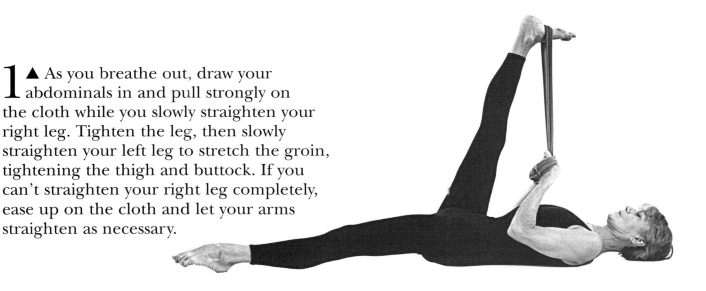

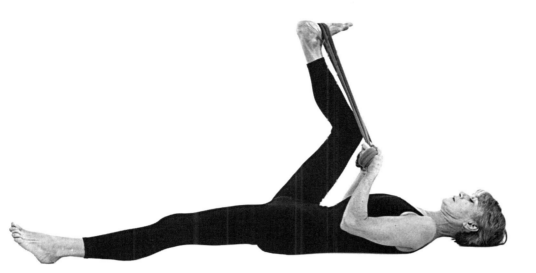

2▲ Breathe normally while you hold, feeling the pull in the back of your leg. Then breathe in as you bend your knee and relax your thigh over your chest.

3 Repeat from step 1 several times, raising the sole of your foot toward the ceiling each time. Then remove the cloth and put your foot on the floor close to your buttocks. Repeat the exercise with your left leg.

Helpful Hints

You may find your legs quiver or shake in this exercise. That just means your muscles are tight. So let your legs shake. As they loosen up, the sensation will eventually disappear.

If your leg leans beyond your hips when it's straight, pull on the cloth more so your lower back doesn't lift. That's harder on your arms but it will strengthen them!

You can increase the stretch once your leg is straight by pulling harder on the cloth, pushing your heel away, or moving the cloth closer to your toes — or, for the maximum stretch, all three.

You can do the exercise with both legs together, but keep the back of your pelvis flat on the floor so your buttocks don't roll up.

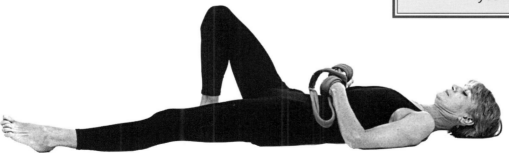

4▲ When you've finished, relax both legs on the floor. Notice how stimulated they feel!

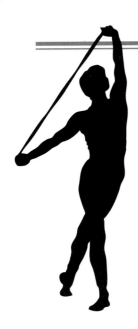

16 Inner Thigh Stretch

In this exercise the cloth supports your legs in the air when they're dropped out to both sides, making it an unusual but relaxed way to stretch your inner thighs.

Cloth length — to suit you

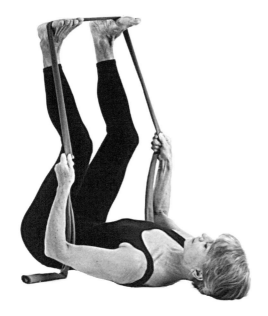

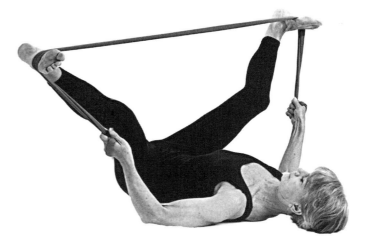

▲ **L**ie on the floor on your back, knees over your chest. Put the middle of the cloth across the soles of your feet, then raise both legs so they're over your hips, bending your knees if necessary.

1 ▲ Let the cloth slip through your hands as you slide your feet along it to each side as far as possible. Circle your hands into the ends once or twice and relax your legs.

3 Stay in this position while you relax your legs as much as you can. Then, with your arms wide, pull on the cloth with your right hand so your right leg lowers toward the floor. Bring your right elbow down to stop you from rolling too far. Then pull with your left hand. Alternate pulling with each hand so your pelvis rocks slowly from side to side. This will increase the stretch to the lowered leg and also gently rotate your lower spine.

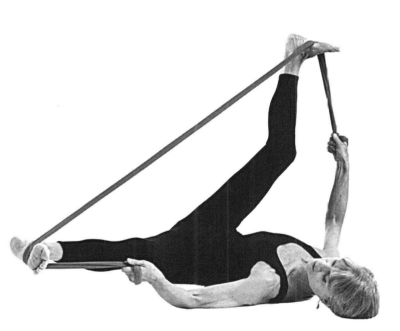

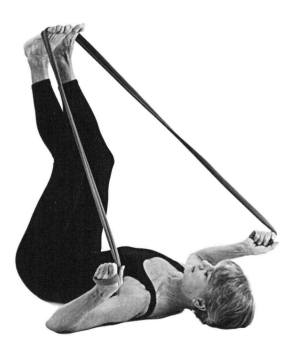

2 ▲ Breathe normally in this stretch and try to relax your whole body. If you're feeling too much pull your legs will tense up, so open them only to the point where they're relaxed, yet still being stretched.

4 ▲ To come out of the stretch, first centre yourself, then pull on both ends of the cloth and slide your feet along it to bring them back over your hips.

5 Bend your knees, remove the cloth, and place your feet, one at a time, on the floor close to your buttocks.

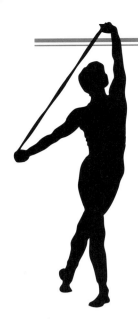

17 Full Body Stretch

In this exercise the stretch comes from lifting your upper body out of your hips while holding your legs and buttocks tight. You may not seem to use the cloth but it helps keep your energy focused in your body, not your hands.

Cloth length — about .6 metre (2 feet)

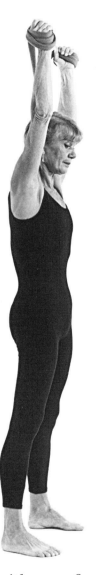

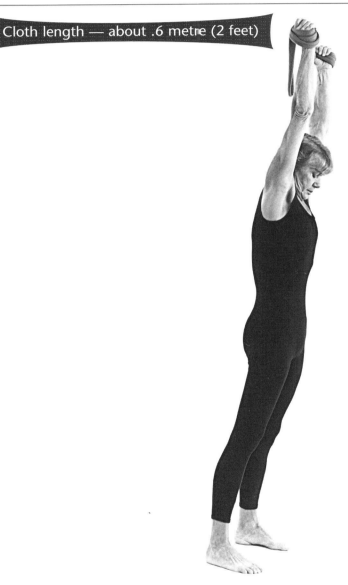

▲ Stand with your feet hip-width apart, toes forward, and arms straight up from your shoulders. If your arms don't go straight up, or if that position pulls your body backward, then slant your arms slightly forward.

1 ▲ Take a deep breath in. *Holding* your breath, lift your arms, shoulders, and shoulder-blades strongly upward, letting your head sink between your shoulders. Tighten your legs and buttocks and press the bottom of your pelvis forward. You should feel your abdominals drawn in and your whole body lengthened.

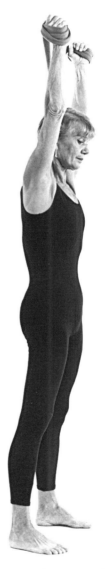

2 ▲ Hold the pull — and your breath — while you feel the stretch through your body, then let your breath out as you lower your shoulders, leaving your arms up, relaxed.

3 Repeat from step 1 several times.

4 When you've finished, bring your arms down and try to maintain the lengthened feeling in your body.

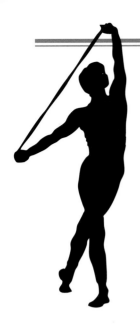

18 Full Spine and Back Stretch

This exercise, like Exercise 1, stretches your neck, spine, and upper back, but here your lower back gets stretched as well. You'll feel a great pull through your whole back.

Cloth length — about 0.6 metre (2 feet)

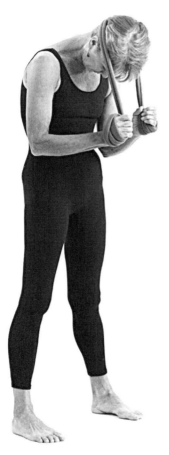

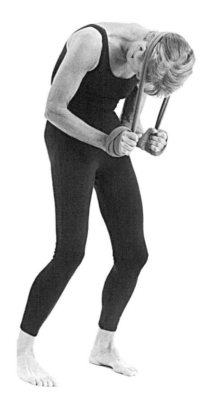

▲ **S**tand with your feet hip-width apart, toes forward, and arms down. Lower your head over your chest until your neck muscles are completely relaxed. Then place the cloth across the back of your head, just above your ears. Lower your hands and relax your shoulders so your hands hang down. Take a deep breath in.

1 ▲ As you breathe out, draw your abdominals in strongly, bend your knees, and press the bottom of your buttocks firmly forward so the length of your spine is completely rounded. Then press down gently on the cloth.

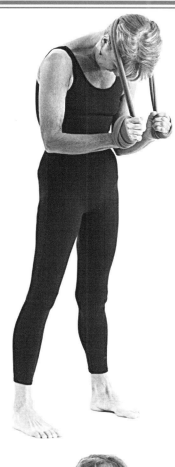

2 ◄ Hold while you feel the stretch as it pulls through your spine and back. Then relax your pull on the cloth, leave your head dropped over, and breathe in as you straighten your legs and back.

3 Repeat from step 1 several times. When you've finished, remove the cloth from your head and straighten up slowly, bringing your head up last.

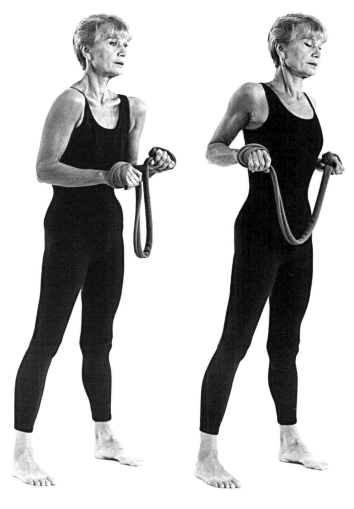

5 ▲▲ Lower your elbows to your sides and circle your shoulders loosely, front to back.

4 ◄ To counteract the stretch, take a deep breath in as you raise your elbows to both sides, shoulder height. Then breathe out as you press your chest forward and your arms back, contracting your shoulderblades.

Helpful Hints

Don't bend your knees so much that there's a strain on your thighs. Bend them only enough to bring your tailbone forward and round your lower back.

When you press down on the cloth, don't lower your body. Instead, think of your head and tailbone pressing toward each other as though to complete a circle, with the stronger pressure coming up from your tailbone.

Don't tighten your shoulders. Either leave them relaxed or press them down to increase the stretch through your upper back.

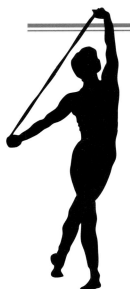

19 Shoulder Stretch

This is a simple but effective exercise for stretching out the tightness that keeps your shoulders lifted. If you do it regularly, you'll soon find that your shoulders are noticeably lower.

Cloth length— at least 1.2 metres (4 feet)

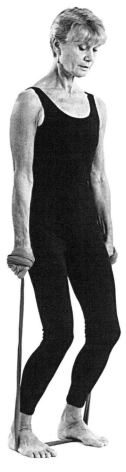

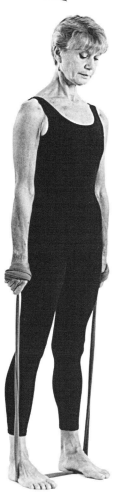

▲ **H**old one end of the cloth in each hand and stand on the middle of it, feet hip-width apart and toes forward. Bend your knees a little and circle your hands into the cloth until it's tight between your hands and feet. Shift your feet to centre the cloth if you need to. Draw your abdominals in and tilt your head forward so your chin is down. Hold the cloth firmly and take a deep breath in.

1 ▲ As you breathe out, keep your abdominals drawn in and your body straight while you slowly straighten your legs. If you can't straighten them, move your feet a little closer together.

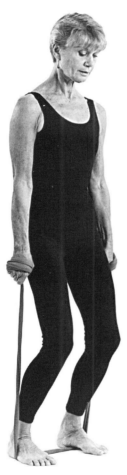

Helpful Hints

If you don't feel a pull in your shoulders, move your feet farther apart to shorten the cloth.

If your back is straight, you should feel a strong pull between your shoulder-blades as well as in your shoulders.

2▲ Stay here as long as you wish, breathing normally while you feel the pull on your shoulders. Then breathe in as you bend your knees.

3 Repeat as often as you wish.

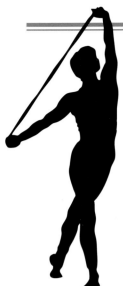

20 Upper Back Contraction

In this exercise the cloth creates a resistance for your back to work against so you can grip the muscles between your shoulder-blades. At the same time you'll feel a stretch in your upper arms, shoulders, and chest.

> Cloth length — 0.75 to 1 metre
> (2-1/2 to 3 feet)

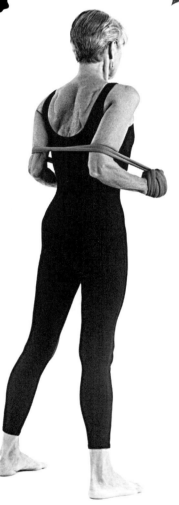

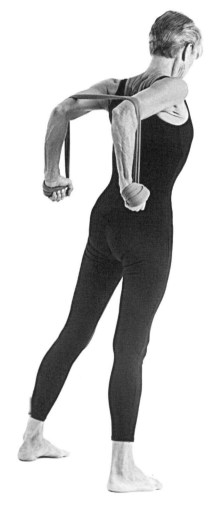

▲ **S**tand with your feet a little wider than hip-width apart, toes forward. Lift the cloth over your head and place it across the back of your arms, just above the elbows. Bring your hands forward, wrists straight and elbows bent at your sides. Take a deep breath in.

1 ▲ As you breathe out, draw your abdominals in, pull your shoulders back, and contract your shoulder-blades. Then press your hands strongly downward behind you, keeping your elbows bent to the back. Tilt your head forward to relax your neck.

If your back is tightly rounded, you will feel little, if any, grip in your upper back. In this case, use the exercise at first simply to loosen it. Emphasize pulling your shoulders back and pressing your chest forward with less backward pressure from your arms.

Be sure your hands press strongly downward as well as back so your shoulders are pulled down. You shouldn't feel any muscles "bunched up" at your neck.

As a further step to add stretch to your spine, pull the top of your head slowly down toward the floor. Try not to tighten your throat.

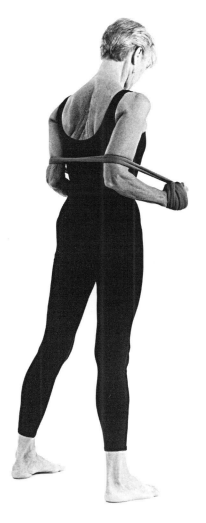

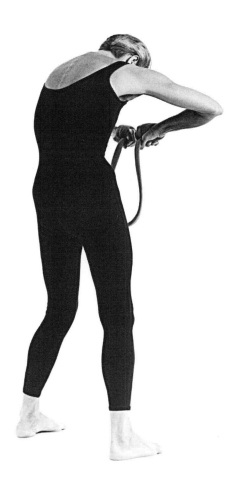

2▲ Hold while you feel the strong pull in your upper back, then breathe in as you relax your muscles.

3 Repeat from step 1 several times.

4▲ When you've finished, bring your arms in front to stretch your back: lower your head and pull your arms and shoulders strongly forward as you round your back and press it out.

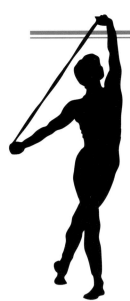

21 Shoulder Rotation

This exercise rolls your shoulders forward, which allows you to put your hand on your back as in Exercise 6. With your arm tightened, it firms the triceps at the back of your upper arm.

Cloth length — about 1 metre (3 feet)

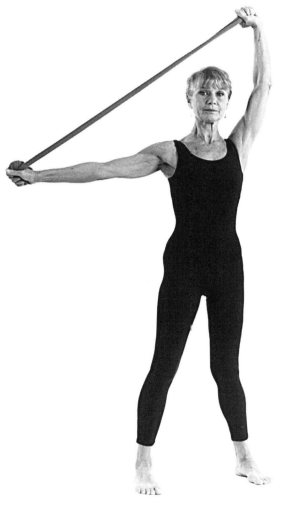

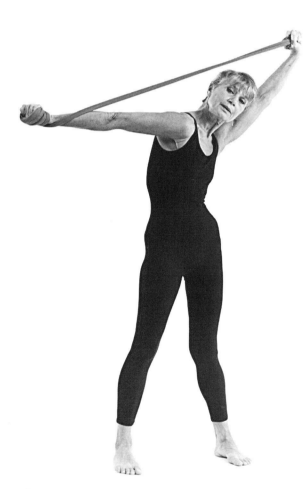

▲ Holding the cloth between your hands stand with your feet a little wider than hip-width apart, toes forward, and abdominals lightly drawn in. Raise your left arm overhead and straighten your right arm to the side at shoulder height, wrist straight. Take a deep breath in. (This exercise can be done sitting or standing.)

1▲ As you breathe out, draw your abdominals in and turn your right hand and arm over, rolling your shoulder forward in the joint. Then tighten your arm.

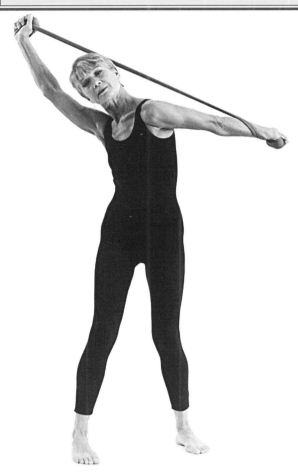

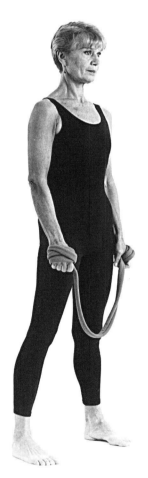

2▲ Breathe in as you lift your shoulder a little to rotate the arm back. Quickly change arms and breathe out as you roll your left shoulder forward. (Or, if it's more comfortable, take your time and breathe as necessary.)

3▲ Alternate sides several times. When you've finished, relax your arms down.

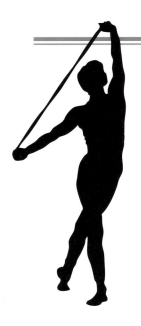

22 Arm Strengthening

This is a simple-looking but powerful exercise for strengthening your arms. It has a strong effect on the shoulder and upper arm muscles as well as those at the sides of your ribs.

Cloth length — about 1 metre (3 feet)

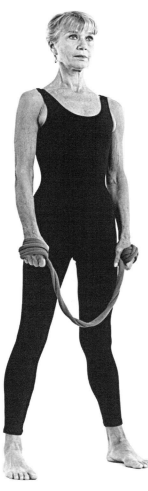

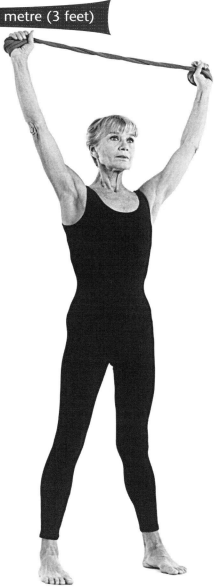

▲ Stand with your feet a little wider than hip-width apart, toes forward, abdominals lightly drawn in, arms down with the cloth between your hands, and back erect. (This exercise can be done sitting or standing.)

1 ▲ Take a deep breath in as you raise your arms overhead, straightening the cloth.

Don't tighten your arms when you pull on the cloth. Keep the energy in your hands pressing out and your shoulders pressing down. This can make your arms shake, especially if they're weak, but that will lessen — or disappear — as your deeper muscles strengthen.

To prevent your back from arching, hold the cloth above your head, not behind it, and be sure to keep your abdominals drawn in. Your body should have a strong "hold" through it.

Your elbows shouldn't come down lower than shoulder height. If they do your shoulders will get pushed up. Focus on pressing your shoulders down and let your elbows bend naturally to come in line with them.

This exercise has a stretching as well as a strengthening effect on your upper arm muscles. To increase both effects, hold the exercise for a longer time count.

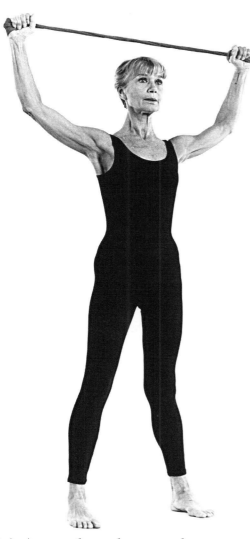

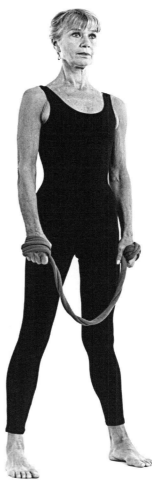

2▲ As you breathe out, draw your abdominals in and pull outward on the cloth as hard as you can. Then press your shoulders down, letting your elbows bend.

3 Hold for a slow count of 3, then breathe in as you lift your arms up, relaxing your shoulders and your pull on the cloth.

4▲ Repeat from step 2 several times. When you've finished, relax your arms down.

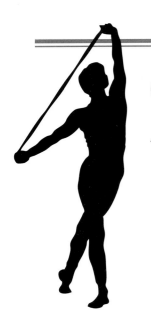

23 Thigh Stretch

This is a great stretch for the quadriceps, the muscles in the front of your thighs. It's usually done by pulling your foot toward your buttocks, which arches the lower back. The way it's done here is safer because it keeps your pelvis straight.

> Cloth length —
> as short as you can make it without arching your back

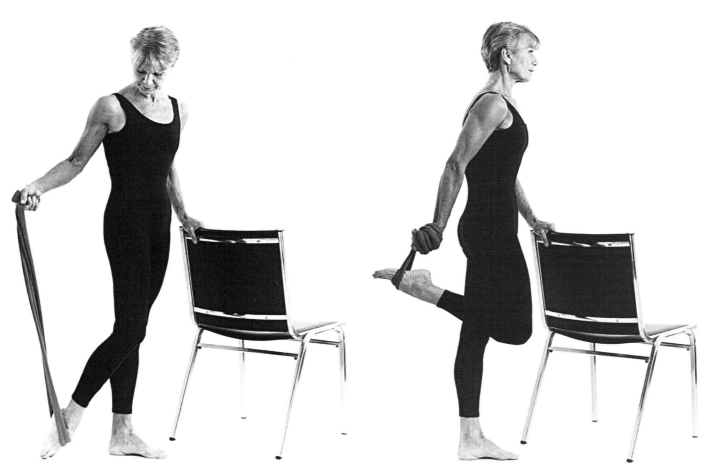

▲ ▲ Stand next to a wall or other support. Hold both ends of the cloth in your right hand, with your hand at your side and slightly behind you. Place your left hand on the support. Hold the cloth so the loop just touches the floor and put your right foot into it, sole facing back. Then circle your hand into the cloth, raising your foot off the floor.* Hold the cloth firmly and take a deep breath in.

*If this position arches your back, bend your supporting knee a little and bring the bottom of your pelvis forward in a "pelvic tilt." If the back of your thigh cramps, straighten your leg and start again.

Make the cloth short enough so the arm holding your foot is straight. That's less tiring than keeping your elbow bent.

If the stretch pulls on your knee, do the exercise more gently.

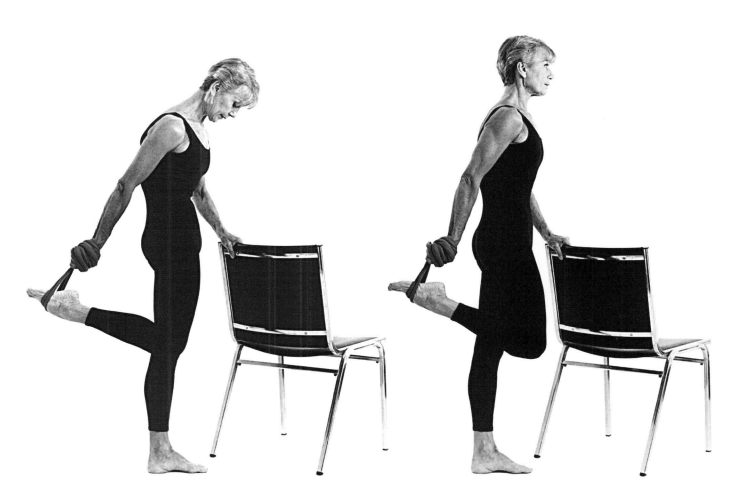

1▲ As you breathe out, draw your abdominals in and tighten your buttocks. Then press the bottom of your pelvis forward and at the same time press your foot down into the loop.

2▲ Hold while you feel the stretch to your thigh, then breathe in as you relax your muscles.

3 Repeat from step 1 several times. When you've finished, change the cloth to your left foot and repeat the exercise.

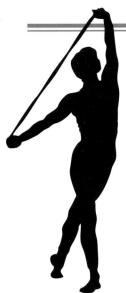

24 Spine Rotation

This exercise rotates your spine and strengthens the muscles around your ribcage as you turn your upper body while holding your hips firmly forward. The feeling is one of tightening an inner coil.

Cloth length — at least 1 metre (3 feet)

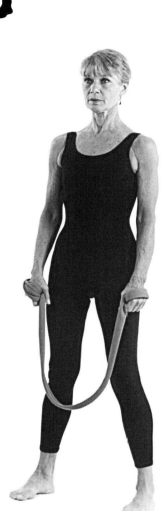

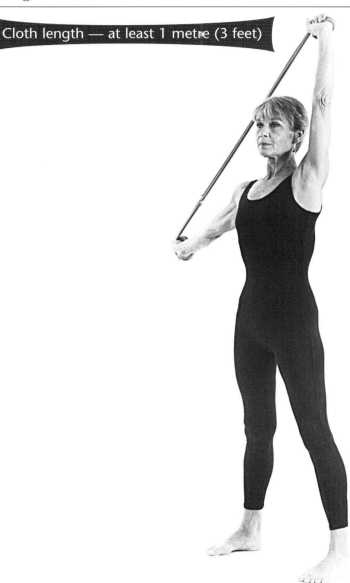

▲ **S**tand with your feet a little wider than hip-width apart, toes forward, abdominals lightly drawn in, and arms down.

1 ▲ Take a deep breath in as you lift your left arm straight up from your shoulder and open your right arm to the side, keeping it low.

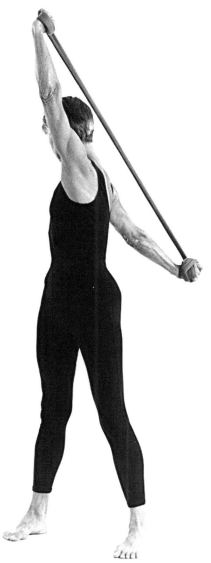

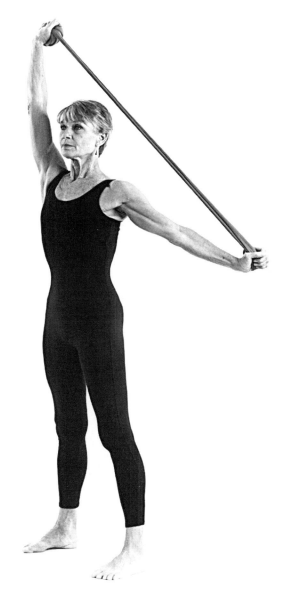

2▲ As you breathe out, draw your abdominals in strongly and tighten your legs. Turn your upper body to the right, pressing your right shoulder down and your right arm around behind you. Let your left arm move with your body.

3▲ Breathe in as you return to face front, reversing your arms, and breathe out as you turn to the left. Turn to both sides several times. Finish facing front and relax your arms down.

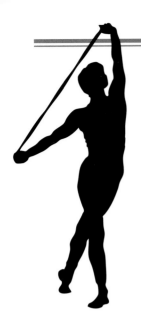

25 Stretching and Strengthening the Torso

Side-bending exercises can put strain on the lower back. This one avoids strain by lifting your weight out of your spine. At the same time it strengthens the deep, skeletal muscles that support your weight and help you to stand tall.

Cloth length — at least 1 metre (3 feet)

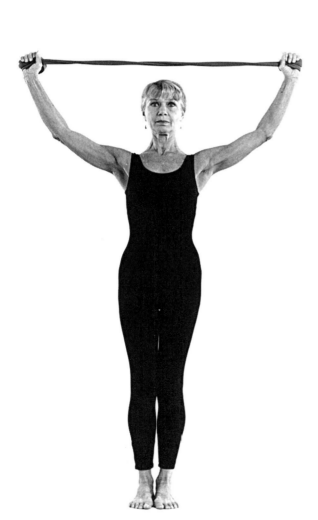

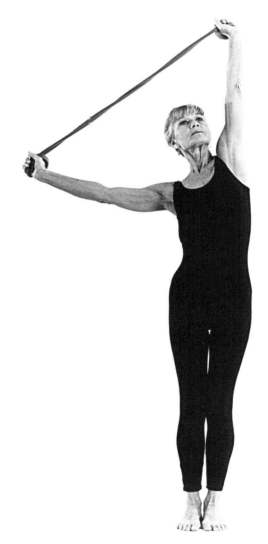

▲ **S**tand with your feet together, toes forward, abdominals drawn in, and back erect. Lift your arms overhead with the cloth straight between your hands.

1▲ Take a deep breath in as you lift your left arm strongly up from the shoulder.

Think of this as a stretch and strength exercise, not as a side bend. As you go from side to side, focus both your mind and energy into the arm that's pulling up. The side arm presses down only to create resistance, which helps lengthen the opposite side while strengthening the internal muscles as the body pulls up.

Keep both arms straight but not tensed and both hands well out from your body. Press the shoulder of the side arm down along with the arm.

You can increase the strengthening effect by holding to the side for a longer time or bending more. If you do this, remember to keep your body pulling up.

3 Breathe in as you pull with your left hand to straighten your body, and in a smooth continuous movement breathe out as you lift your right arm up and press down with the left.

4 Alternate slowly from side to side, feeling the stretch in your lengthened side while your inner muscles pull you upward.

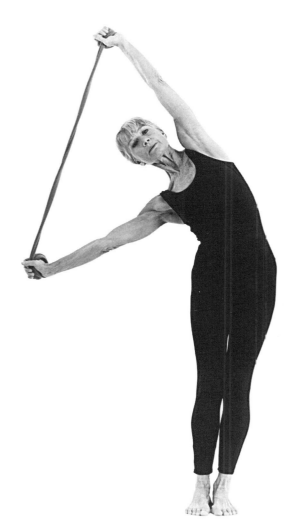

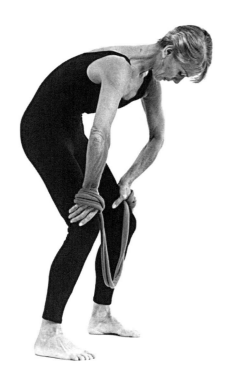

2▲ As you breathe out, lift your shoulder higher and at the same time press your right arm slowly toward the floor. Keep pressing your arm down until you feel the stretch through your left side all the way down to your hip-bone.

5▲ When you've finished, separate your feet and place your hands on your thighs. Draw your abdominals in, round your lower back, and gently press out through the back of your waist.

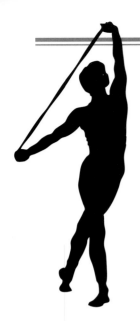

26 Lower Back Stretch (2)

This is a good exercise to do to relieve any kinks in your lower back. It gives a stronger stretch to the back of your waist than Exercise 9.

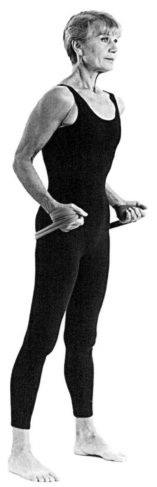

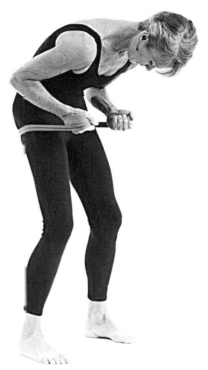

▲ Hold one end of the cloth in each hand, with the loop touching the floor. Step over the loop and space your feet a little wider than hip-width apart, toes forward. Circle your hands into the cloth until it's up across your tailbone, then bring your hands forward, elbows bent at your sides. Take a deep breath in.

1 ▲ As you breathe out, draw your abdominals in strongly, bend your knees, and bring your tailbone forward, rounding your lower back. Then lower your head and pull the cloth forward with your hands, gradually increasing the pressure.

If your abdominals "grip," you'll tense up and stop breathing. Make sure you draw them in and breathe out continuously. The more strongly you pull your abdominals toward your spine while pressing your hands forward, the more stretch you'll feel in your lower back.

To increase the stretch to either side of your lower back, keep the pressure on your tailbone and alternately straighten one leg while bending the other knee more.

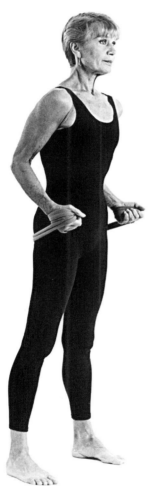

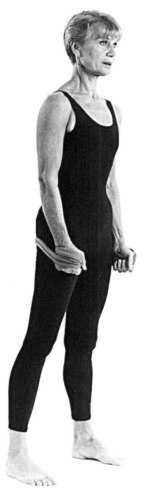

2▲ Hold while you feel the stretch through your lower back, then breathe in as you relax the pull on the cloth and slowly bring yourself up.

3▲ Repeat from step 1 several times. Then relax your arms down.

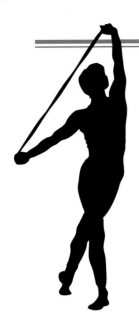

27 Total Body Relaxation

Finish each of your sessions with this wonderfully relaxing "non-exercise." You don't need the cloth and there is nothing to press or pull. Just "hang loose" and let gravity do the rest.

Cloth Length — about 0.6 metre (2 feet)

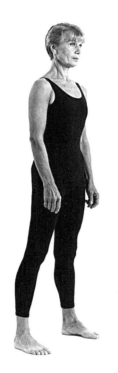

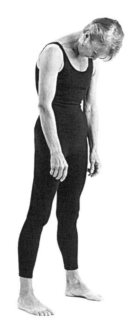

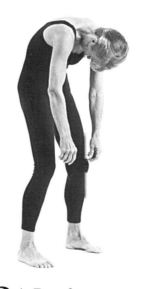

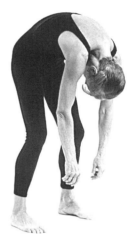

▲ 1 Stand with your feet hip-width apart, toes forward, and your arms relaxed at your sides.

2▲ Lower your head slowly over your chest until your neck muscles are completely relaxed.

3▲ Bend your knees a little, draw your abdominals in lightly, and relax your shoulders forward so your arms dangle in front of your legs.

4▲ Keeping your buttocks forward, lower your head slowly toward the floor until your back is completely rounded and your hands are level with your shins. Pull your arms gently toward the floor, then let them relax. Feel the weight of your arms, head, and back as they hang down. Stay here as long as you wish, letting all tension drain away.

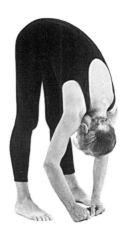

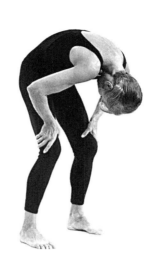

5▲ Now, slowly straighten your legs, letting your body drop further if that happens naturally. Feel the stretch through the back of your legs while the weight of your body hangs from your hips.

6▲▶ When you're ready to come up, lift yourself a little as you bend your knees and place your hands above them. Bring your hips forward over your feet, then walk your hands up your thighs as you slowly straighten your spine, bringing your head up last.

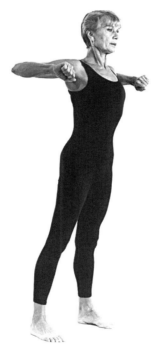

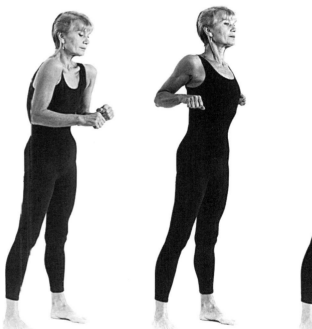

7▲ Take a last deep breath as you raise your elbows to both sides, shoulder height. Then breathe out as you press your chest forward and your arms back, contracting your shoulder blades.

8▲▲▲ Lower your elbows to your sides and circle your shoulders loosely, front to back. Then relax your arms at your sides.

9Enjoy the feeling!

Acknowledgements

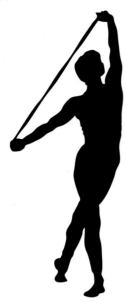

A great many people have passed through my classes since I began teaching in 1978. Little did they — or I — know they were co-creators of a method for well-being that was taking its time to come to fulfilment. Their bodies, problems, and questions brought forth answers and insights that I would not otherwise have known how to explain or verbalize. To all, I say thank you, with special thanks to those who in recent years have encouraged me to "get my ideas out" and, in my sometimes despairing times, have sustained me with their enthusiasm for my work. It has made the years of waiting for the "right time" worthwhile.

I wish to give special thanks here, too, to Shelley Robertson, past editor of the *Toronto Star*, for getting me started on writing about my method with an article in 1981 and, following this, an exercise series in 1985. It was the response to that series that encouraged me to start writing a book, and I remain grateful to Shelley, and to her husband Peter, for their support and friendship over these many years.

I would also like to express my gratitude to Eleanor Johnston for her concern and thoughtfulness in arranging through Paul Madaule the initial contact with my publisher, Ed Boyce. Without their aid, this long awaited project would no doubt have remained only an idea in my head.

The many hours needed to complete the writing of this book would not have been possible without my daughter's assistance in teaching classes for me over these past months. It has been a godsend, and I am not only grateful for her so willing and enthusiastic help but also immensely gratified that my concepts have now become a mainstay for her own life. Thank you Meredith for taking over, and for your love and continuing support.

My thanks to Iris Hamilton, Ann O'Hara, and the others unknown to me who took the time to try out the test kit and report on it. Their input was most helpful in producing the final guidelines.

Sincere thanks to my editors along the way, Pam Harrison, Liz McLeod, and Fiona Mackenzie King, for steering me through uncharted waters with such generous and forgiving patience. Also, thanks to all the seen and unseen people who have worked on this book with Moulin Publishing. Warm thanks go to Andrew Oxenham, also a former dancer with the National Ballet, who has enhanced this book with his excellent photography.

Special mention and thanks are due also to Margaret and Chris Boyce, who unravelled the complexities of incorporating the Stretchcloth into the book and coordinated the many aspects of production.

My deepest thanks are reserved for Ed Boyce and Moulin Publishing for "walking in where angels fear to tread." Thank you, Ed, for your faith in me, and for believing in my "message." May this be not an end, but a new beginning.

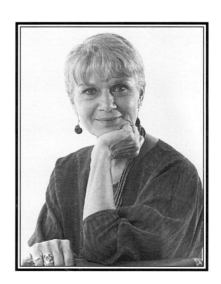